You Hold The Key

You Hold The Key

Your contemplative guide to
unlocking your inner wisdom

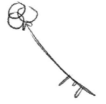

Anna Hei-Ming Resnick

You Hold The Key

Copyright © 2020 by Anna Resnick

Writing and illustrations by Anna Resnick

Published by Anna Resnick
www.intentionallyanna.com

First Edition: December 2020

ISBN: 978-1-7363888-8-4

Dedicated to:

Life
(which includes all the
people, places, and events
that led me here ♡)

Eternally grateful for the One source ☺

How This Book Manifested

I had a vision of the cover page of this book even before I had written a single page. Ever since that insight I let inspiration take the reigns, allowing my heart's inner wisdom spill out the words. There were times when I'd write 40 pages in one setting and weeks where I'd write nothing at all. The process of surrendering to aliveness and letting the book unfold itself was both humbling and exciting. Since none of the writing was forced, making this book was practically effortless.

I intentionally hand-wrote and hand-drew every page to convey the raw messages most directly to you as they were happening. This is my gift to you, from my heart to yours. I hope it fills you up with as much love as it filled me with in its creation.

♡ Anna

How To Read This Book

I first want to clarify – no, there is no one "right" way to read this book; however, if you're wanting to make the most out of this read and don't know where to start, I invite you to read one to two pages either in the morning or at night which are the most potent times. Each page is simple yet reflective, so I'd give each time to marinate overnight for a fuller experience. Reading the right page at the right time is meant to help you heal or recognize a part of yourself that you might've forgotten was there.

With that being said, there are so many subtle differences between you and me that the way this book serves you best might surprise me! Whether you choose to use this book the way I suggested, as an oracle, or something you open every now and then,

✳ simply follow your intuition ✳

(That's the whole point after-all)

♡ Anna

Introduction

In 2nd grade I spent most of my recesses alone in Mrs. Anderson's classroom making books. I remember when I finished "The Piano," a book Mrs. Anderson proudly placed on her shelf for the other students to read. She gifted me an expensive set of gel pens and told me that someday I was going to make a fantastic author.

Three years later my dream was crushed when I failed to make the top three in my 5th grade class's story competition. My mentors warned me that unless I was a Pablo Picasso, I wouldn't make it as an artist. They told me that in reality most artists go broke and become homeless.

In this new "reality" I learned that passions and work were two separate things — work was a means to an end, a vehicle for material wealth. Only until you acquired enough money and success could you celebrate and indulge in your passions.

Instead of pursuing an artistic career I gave in to society's hierarchial structure, relinquishing control over

Introduction

my body and mind to do what others would find respectable. I finally "made it" when I landed a Software Engineering gig at Facebook. Everything I'd spent the last decade working towards was suddenly right at my fingertips, yet I'd still come home after work feeling an emptiness, this deep lack within myself. Surrounded by everything I thought I "should" want made me even more distressed that I was unhappy.

My body rebelled from boredom and constant burn-out cycles. Rather than nurture myself I pushed harder. 'Why was my body such a failure? Why was it broken?' What followed were doctor visits, one illness after another, and lots. of. fear.

I ultimately hit a breaking point, realizing that if I continued on the path that I was on my body would eventually fail me. What would be the point of wealth and success if I died before I ever got to enjoy it?

My body's meltdown was really a demand to stop

Introduction

giving away my power and to finally give into my heart. I instantly dropped everything. I gave up my career, the years I spent working towards my degree, the prestige, the familiarity, and (most difficult) the idea that I needed to be something for someone else.

The next chapter of my life that followed is too complex to simplify in this introduction, but what I can tell you is that is was very magical. Some of the craziest and most eye-opening experiences — living in an RV on a horse ranch, starting a Life Coaching business, presenting workshops to over 500 individuals, nourishing myself back to health, and discovering the sweet spot of work and passion. It was an absolute rollercoaster of highs and lows.

Now having tasted freedom, I don't forsee myself willingly going back to my old prison. Once you get a whiff of what freedom feels like nothing else compares.

Reflecting back to my old self I wondered why it was

Introduction

so difficult to escape, to BE free.

The truth: society's "reality" conditions us our whole lives to NOT be. General society tells you just to do, to succeed by doing and completely ignore your soul, the wise, creative part of you.

During my dark days exploring my shadows, what kept me going and believing in myself were books, words of inspiration, and beautiful images that spoke to my heart. That is also everything this book encapsulates — all the words that kept me moving, believing, dreaming, listening, understanding, and remembering who I am at the end of the day.

Every page of this book has words that resonate deeply with my heart. I've left out all the fluff — only real, raw words of love remain. Some words are tough to swallow, but just like love, the truth isn't always easy to digest. It is, however, always there to protect you and remind you of how worthy you are.

Introduction

Somehow after all these years since 2nd grade I'm back to making books again. As I've found, dreams don't fade; rather, they expand overtime. That little voice in your heart only amplifies as time goes on and it's there for a reason. My question is— are you ready to listen?

♡ Anna

Content

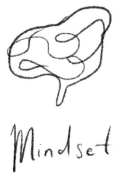

Mindset

What got you

here

will not get you

there

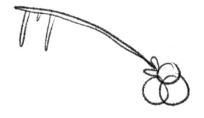

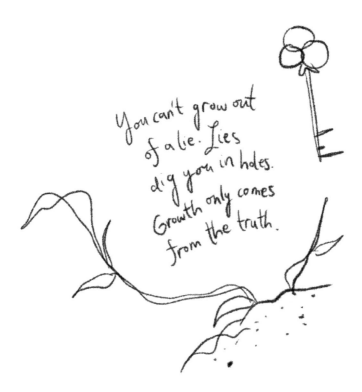

You can't grow out of a lie. Lies dig you in holes. Growth only comes from the truth.

Mindset

What you
see in others
is a reflection
of yourself

You can't spot
what you don't
already know

The darkness
in others is the
darkness you've
seen in yourself

The light in
others is the
light you have
within yourself

How you judge/love
others is how you judge/love
yourself

4

Mindset

Every minute of every day you are dying

When are you going to start living?

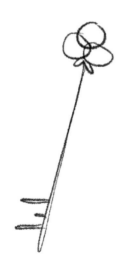

Mindset

You were born into a world
that flooded you with information
on how you "should" be

How you "should"
speak

How you "should"
act

How you "should"
think

And you've become an adaptable actor!

But, the show is over.

You can slip out of that heavy costume

Remove the heavy weight

to let yourself

finally

breathe.

A lot of people get stuck theorizing, planning, and rationalizing how to get from point A to point B

When all it takes is one step

After enough "one steps" in the right direction, how can you not get there?

Mindset

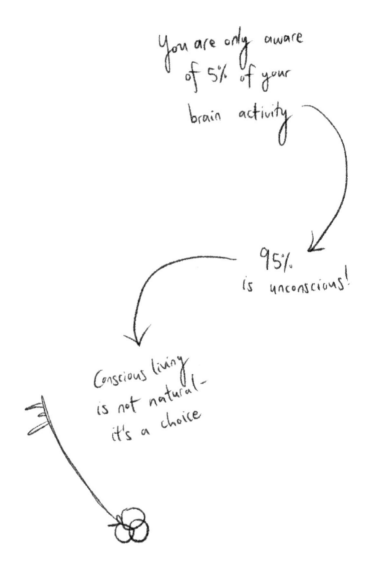

You are only aware of 5% of your brain activity

95% is unconscious!

Conscious living is not natural — it's a choice

Mindset

Awareness is always
the first step, because
how can you change
something that you
are not even fully
conscious of?

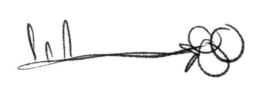

Mindset

You attract who you
are being. When you
are playing a persona
you thus attract people
who amplify
that persona, making
it harder to break
free to find who
you truly are.

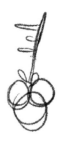

Mindset

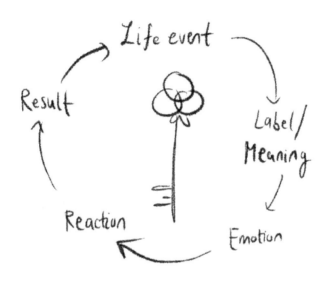

You affect the results in
your life

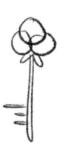

You are
quite literally
spaciousness.
Your body is made
up of atoms that
consist of mostly
~~empty~~ space.

So, when you're feeling small
or constricted you can try to
breathe into the spaciousness
in your body that already
exists.

Rules are made
by humans
and thus
are imperfect.

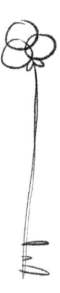

Mindset

Just because you don't
understand it doesn't mean
it isn't true.

Think of all the times
your mind was blown.

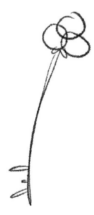

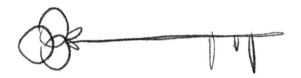

The only moment
that exists is this
moment right now.
Time doesn't stop
for anyone.

Mindset

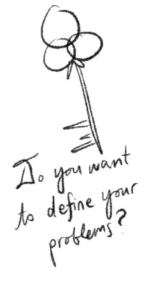

Do you want to define your problems?

Or, do you want your problems to define you?

There is no in between.

Mindset

What you resist
is what you receive....
    for resistance is
    working around a
    "problem"...
       and working around
       a problem makes
       the problem more significant

      whereas...
confronting what you resist
allows you to dissolve
    the problem completely.

Mindset

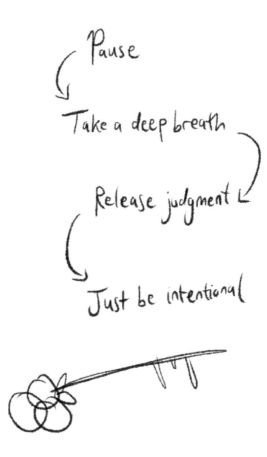

Pause

Take a deep breath

Release judgment

Just be intentional

Mindset

You have ~60,000 thoughts
in a day and ~80%
are negative. Rather than
listen to the pessimistic mind,
tune into your body + heart.
They are much wiser guides.

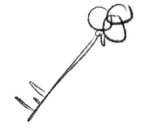

Mindset

Every new path
you carve for
   yourself you also carve

for others as
an alternative
they can take.

You make space
for others simply
by making space
for yourself.

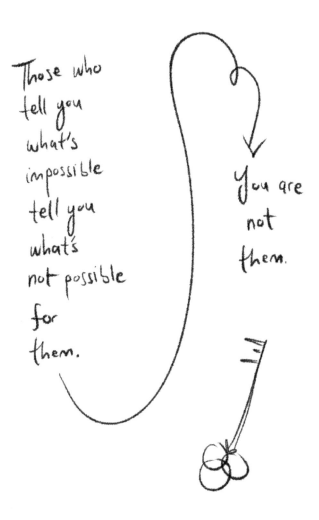

Those who
tell you
what's
impossible
tell you
what's
not possible
for
them.

You are
not
them.

Mindset

Finding balance in life is like holding a steering wheel

If you hold on too tight you'll jolt left and right

If you unconsciously let go you might crash

But, if you release your tension and stay consciously aware you can actually enjoy the ride.

The loudest voices
aren't the most
right, they're just
loud

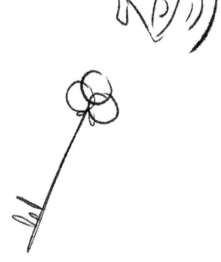

Less is more

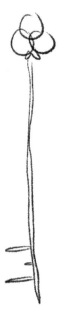

Confidence is
quiet

Mindset

It takes courage
to step out of the
mold and shape
yourself.

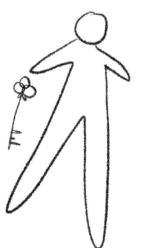

No one can tell
you what to think or
feel — no one can
control your mind.

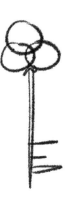

Mindset

Question the
person that
tells you <u>not</u>
to question.

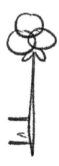

Mindset

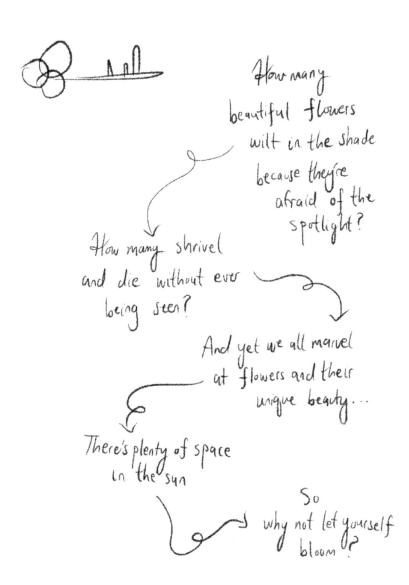

How many
beautiful flowers
wilt in the shade
because they're
afraid of the
spotlight?

How many shrivel
and die without ever
being seen?

And yet we all marvel
at flowers and their
unique beauty...

There's plenty of space
in the sun

So
why not let yourself
bloom?

No label can
fully encapsulate
the beauty and
complexity of
you.

Mindset

You immediately put
ointment over a cut,
yet you brush a negative
feeling to the side. Your
mind created your impatience
to trip and fall, yet you
only treat your physical scar.
What would <u>actually</u> be
the cure?

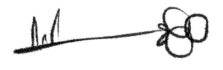

Mindset

Not taking action
is an action.
It's the action
of inaction.

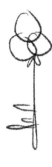

Mindset

What are you
waiting for?
The perfect moment
doesn't exist.

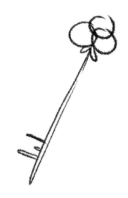

Mindset

Sure, you can go through all of the
"what if you fail" hypotheticals,
but you can just as well go
through all of the
"what if you suceed" hypotheticals.
They're all just thoughts anyways.

Form deep ~~attachments~~

connections

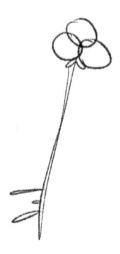

If not you, then <u>who</u>?

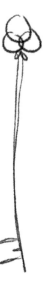

If not now, then <u>when</u>?

Mindset

Your energy isn't linear.
Rest, creation, and rejuvenation
come in waves. You can let
yourself flow with it.

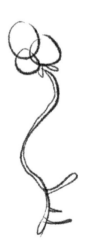

Mindset

You can't defeat a problem at the same level of consciousness that was used to create the problem.

Mindset

What you focus on
is what you create.

⟶ If you focus on the
problem you create
more of the problem.

⟶ If you focus on the
solution you create
the solution.

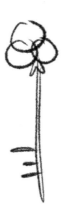

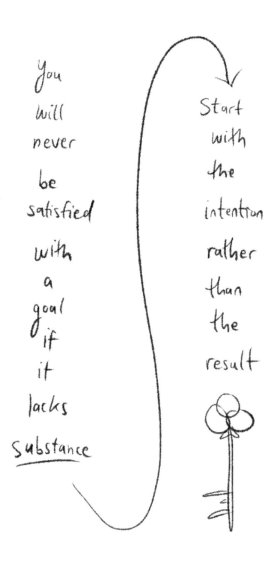

You will never be satisfied with a goal if it lacks substance

Start with the intention rather than the result

Mindset

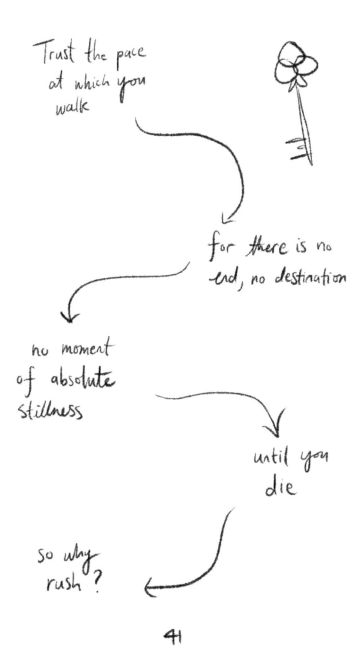

Trust the pace
at which you
walk

for there is no
end, no destination

no moment
of absolute
stillness

until you
die

so why
rush?

Mindset

There will always be things "to do" even on your deathbed, so why spend your whole life stressing over this imagined list?

You don't become "good" by ridding yourself of "bad" qualities, but rather by finding the goodness already within you and allowing it to emerge.

Mindset

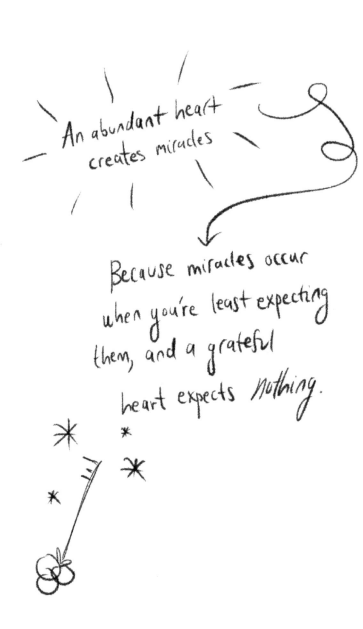

An abundant heart
creates miracles

Because miracles occur
when you're least expecting
them, and a grateful
heart expects *nothing*.

You don't know
what you don't know,
so how do you know
that you know?

Mindset

~ 95% of your thoughts
today are your thoughts
from yesterday. Your
mind clings onto the past.
So, if you feel like your
thoughts are stuck in
a loop, they are.
To get out of the loop you
must get out of your
head.

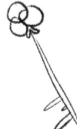

Mindset

Everyone is winging it. Some people are just great pretenders.

Mindset

Instant gratification
from Amazon Prime, Grubhub, Netflix,
and other similar innovations
make you believe
that "life should be easy"

Life shouldn't be anything —
life is just life.

Addictive Habits

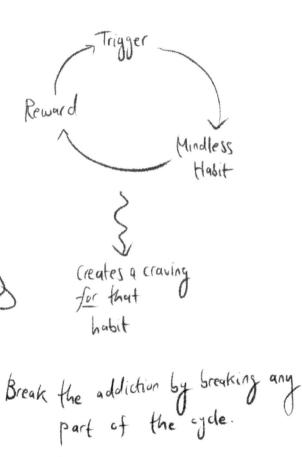

Trigger

Reward

Mindless Habit

Creates a craving for that habit

Break the addiction by breaking any part of the cycle.

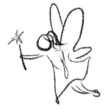

If a fairy could magically
poof away your 3 greatest
pains in life right now, what
would you be doing?

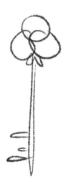

For every
disempowered
thought,
what are
3 honest empowered
thoughts you can
try on (just for today)?

Mindset

Anything you crave
you can create

Because what you're
searching for is not
a person or a thing

But rather,
a feeling

And, there are many,
many ways to create
a feeling.

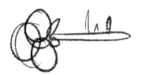

Mindset

Your "what is" is
keeping you from
your "what can be."

What do you want more?

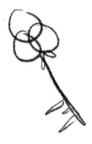

Mindset

You only have the perspective of your vantage point.

Other vantage points paint a completely different world.

And each perspective is necessary to have the whole picture.

Openness, not constriction, creates unity

A one-size-fits all solution makes no sense. We all have uniquely different needs.

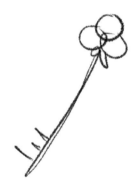

Mindset

All emotion comes from these three forces:

Body
language

Thoughts
you're telling
yourself — General
focus

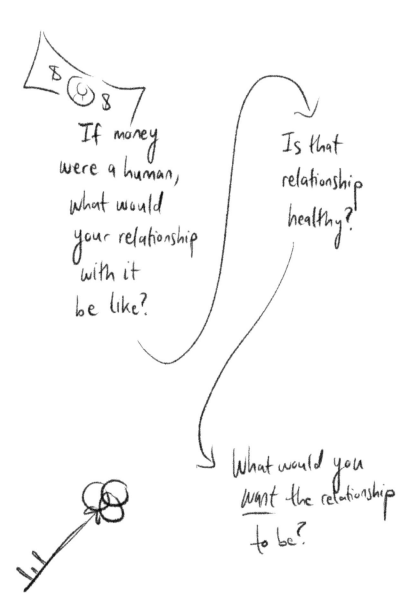

If money were a human, what would your relationship with it be like?

Is that relationship healthy?

What would you want the relationship to be?

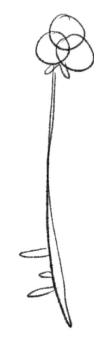

How do you
want to be remembered?
As the person that
gave into your fears
or as the person that
gave into your heart?

So you might as well
show up fully
as you.

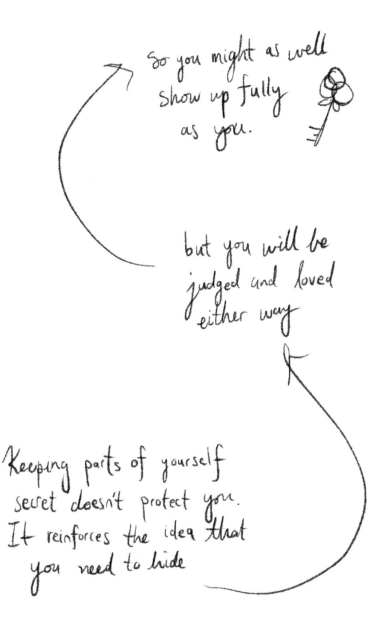

but you will be
judged and loved
either way

Keeping parts of yourself
secret doesn't protect you.
It reinforces the idea that
you need to hide

Mindset

Opening your
heart doesn't
make you
vulnerable
unless you're
expecting
something
in return

but expecting
something in
return isn't
really love,
is it?

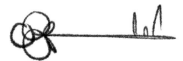

Mindset

No one knows you
more than you.

So, why do you think
they know better what
you need to do?

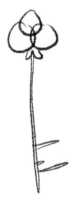

Mindset

You don't get to decide all of what happens to you, but you do get to decide how you react.

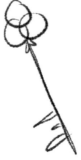

Mindset

Failure is inevitable.

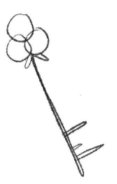

Happiness is optional.

Mindset

It's the idea that
life must not be
messy that's driving
you insane
(not the
mess itself)

Because
life is messy

And, a little
bit of dirt
isn't going to
kill you.

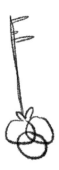

Describing a color to the colorblind
is not the same as actually
seeing it

You can't possibly know
the full depth of an experience
unless you've actually tried it.

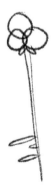

Mindset

On the other side of fear
is freedom

Pain Body

Pain Body

At the end of the day
everyone just wants
to be happy

Happiness is a
feeling that you
can't see

Why then do you
assume that anyone
is any happier?

Pain Body

You aren't superhuman
and you don't need to be.

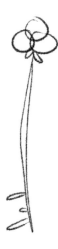

Pain Body

You are way more than your
age
race
hair
height
face
name
paycheck
job title
car
nose
weight

None of that is you; none of that
defines you.

Pain Body

What's broken down
can be built up again.
The fact that you
created it in the
first place means you
have the power to
create it again.

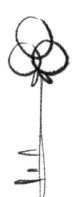

Pain Body

It's okay to not be okay.

If
everything
was
easy
and
always
went
right,
then
what
would
be
the
point
of
anything
?

Any overreaction is a
sign to look
within.

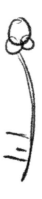

Pain Body

Your feelings
are always
valid . . .

because if you're
sad, who can
say that
you're not?

That simply would
not make sense.

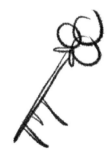

Those who judge
what you do are
really judging themselves
for what they do.

Pain Body

You are doing the best
you can with what
you have

and so is
everyone else.

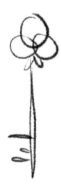

Pain Body

Labels/identities trap you
into a box that was
never there to begin with.

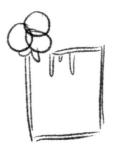

Your mistakes and failures won't make-or-break the right relationships. The right people will love you as you are.

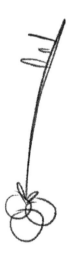

There will
always be
someone that
already has
what you want,
and there will
always be someone
that wants what
you already
have.

You can always make
space for yourself.

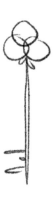

Love doesn't blind you.

Fear does.

Pain Body

Fear creates walls

Walls keep everyone out

you put up a wall when you distrust yourself around others

Love creates boundaries

Boundaries allow the right people in

you define a boundary when you honor yourself and what you need

Pain Body

Why intentionally speak to ears that aren't trying to hear you?

It's essentially talking to thin air, but at least air doesn't judge you.

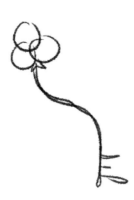

84

Pain Body

Everything can be broken
down into bite-sized
chunks. If it's still
too large,
keep cutting.

Pain Body

What's the next
best feeling you
can have right now?
What's the next
immediate step you
can take?

Pain Body

Some of life's
best natural
medicines:

→ sunlight
→ water
→ laughter
→ tears
→ herbs
→ deep breaths
→ fresh air
→ love

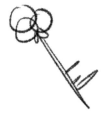

Pain Body

What happened happened for you.

↳ What's happening is meant to happen.

↳ What will happen will happen as it should.

There are no mistakes in the timing of your life.

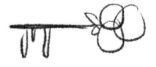

Pain Body

If you removed the
empty space from our
atoms, all 7 billion
of us humans would
fit into a sugar
cube

You are not meant to
be tight and constricted
you are
open and spacious

What's the worst that can happen?

Is it death?

... or is it a story?

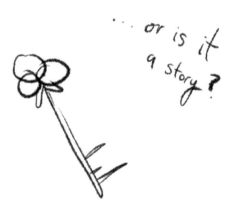

Pain Body

You deserve to feel what you feel.
It doesn't always
have to be about someone
or something.

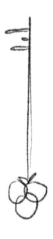

Pain Body

Catching yourself in a spiral
means you're already out of it.
It's judgment that sucks you
back in.

You can start over
as many times
as you need.

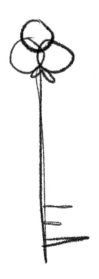

Pain Body

Who is it that
you are still seeking
validation, authority, or
safety from?

What does that person
offer that you think
you can't give to
yourself?

Pain Body

No
matter
how
thin

you
slice
it

There
will
always
be
two
sides.

Pain Body

If you are going
to blame others
for your problems,
then at least blame
them <u>fully</u>

"I blame you for all the
shit you put me through"

<u>and</u>

"I blame you for making
me as strong and resilient
as I am today"

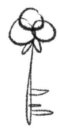

Pain Body

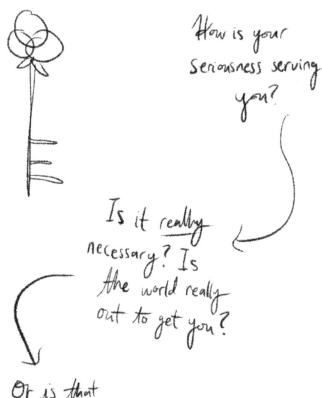

How is your
Seriousness serving
you?

Is it really
necessary? Is
the world really
out to get you?

Or is that
just what you've
been told?

Drop what
isn't yours.

It's okay to need
to be held. It's okay
to ask for space to
simply be seen and
listened to. It's okay
to have these needs —
we all do.

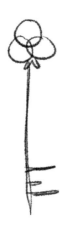

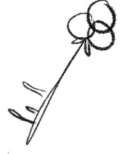

Competition doesn't birth creativity, it suffocates it.

Your voice and unique experiences matter.

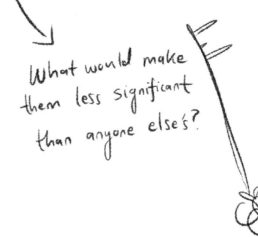

What would make them less significant than anyone else's?

It's not your job to
make someone else
happy.

Your only obligation is
to yourself.

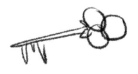

Pain Body

This feeling
will pass.
You are never
stuck.

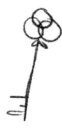

Pain Body

Forgiveness
is
for giving

it's giving to
yourself and
everyone else
involved

and having
the mature
perspective to
see that

no one is the enemy

Pain Body

We tend to think things
could've been better.
The truth is, they could've
been worse too.

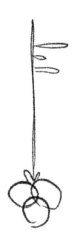

If you were
your close friend,
what advice
would you
give yourself?

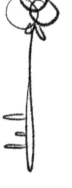

Pain Body

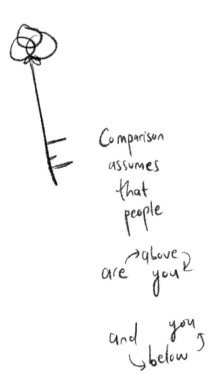

Comparison
assumes
that
people

are →above↗ you?

and you↘ below↙

When we're all on the same level

Pain Body

Everyone poops.

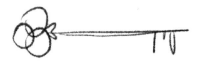

Pain Body

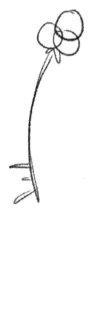

Fear is what makes
you both human
and brave.

There is no
courage without
fear

Pain Body

No one needs to be
"saved" by you.

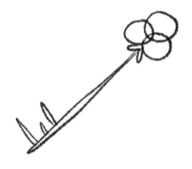

No one is
broken.

Pain Body

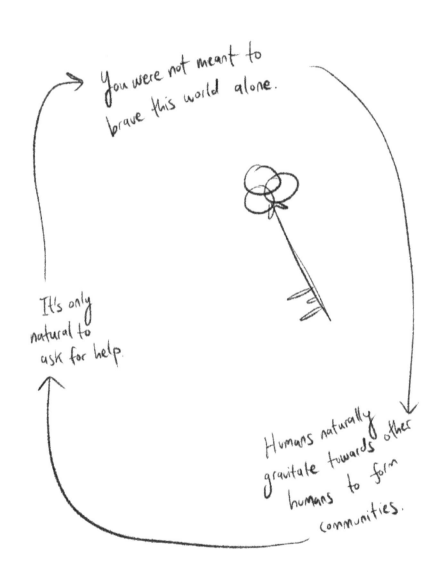

You were not meant to brave this world alone.

It's only natural to ask for help.

Humans naturally gravitate towards other humans to form communities.

Pain Body

Anxiety is in the anticipation
of an event that hasn't yet
happened, which is the
safest part!

Pain Body

When you're feeling low, give
yourself the space to actually
be with that feeling. Don't
judge it. Acknowledge it.
Understand it. Make friends
with it. And it will pass a
lot quicker than you'd
expect.

Pain Body

Just like with any phase,
this phase feels never-ending...
but also just like with any
phase, this phase <u>will</u> end.

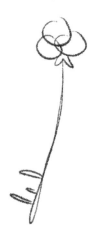

Pain Body

There's nothing you need
to prove because you
are already enough.

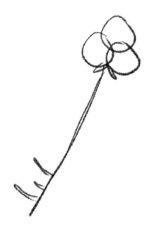

Pain Body

No

You can't pick out
the parts of me you
don't like and tear me
apart.

I am to be devoured

whole

or not at all.

Best Medicine For Anger

→ Screaming in the car

→ Writing an unfiltered letter
    and then burning it

→ Punching a pillow

→ 15 jumping jacks

→ Stomping on the ground

→ Ripping up recycled paper

→ Sprinting across the park

→ Angry crying

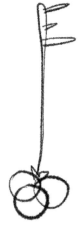

Pain Body

You can't change someone's mind
about you if their mind is
already made.

Someone that isn't willing to see
your heart isn't worth your time.

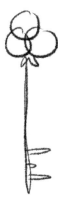

Pain Body

So much of the weight
you are carrying isn't
yours

Drop what isn't needed
anymore and life
becomes much
lighter

Strong and sensitive
are not opposites.

It takes strength
to be vulnerable.

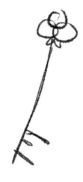

Pain Body

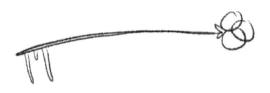

There's no better stress relief
than a good cry.

Let it all out.

Let it all go.

Allow the
flow.

Pain Body

Discomfort in your body
is a signal to
check your emotional
state. Stay curious.

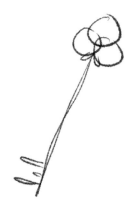

Pain Body

Comparing yourself
to someone else's
highlight reel doesn't
make sense. Life is a
myriad of shots —
most of which you
don't see. Why
scale your life
according to the most
unrealistic depiction
of it?

Pain Body

The only reason
I speak so
directly to you
is because
I've had your
thoughts too.
You're not alone.

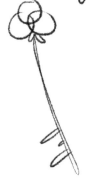

Pain Body

What would it feel like to think all
of the things you "shouldn't" think
and to blurt out all the words
you "shouldn't" say?

Why not try it
when no one's around?

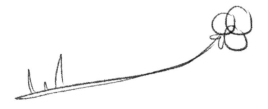

Pain Body

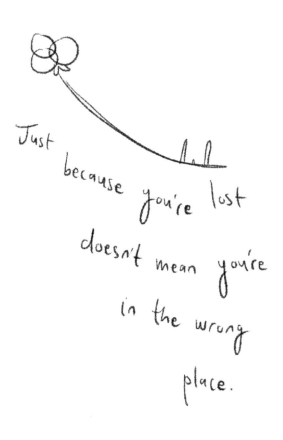

Just because you're lost doesn't mean you're in the wrong place.

Pain Body

Striving to be
real rather than
perfect makes
life much simpler.
It makes life what
it actually is.

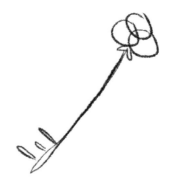

Pain Body

A tornado will rip
apart a house, yet
leave a small blade
of grass unscathed.

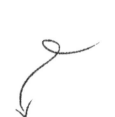

What's the
difference between
the two?

One tries to stand
strong and fight
while the other bends
over and lets the
storm pass.

Some battles don't
need to be fought
to be won.

No one looks at a
butterfly and thinks—
'Dammit, why were
you ever a caterpillar?'

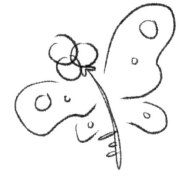

because we
know the caterpillar
phase was a
necessary part
of the transition
(and caterpillars
are uniquely
interesting)

So why is it
that you look
back at your
old phases with
such distaste and
regret?

Pain Body

You're doing your best, and there's nothing better than that.

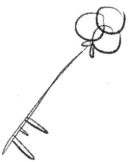

If you really wish to
    be someone else
then you must
give up friends,
family, belongings
you have acquired

too.

Now is that still
what you want
    to do?

Pain Body

What's left unsaid may
say more than what
words can.

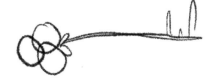

Everything is made up of
tiny steps

Every
tiny step
is significant.

Pain Body

One deep breath.

That's all it takes.

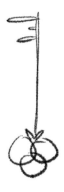

Awakening

Awakening

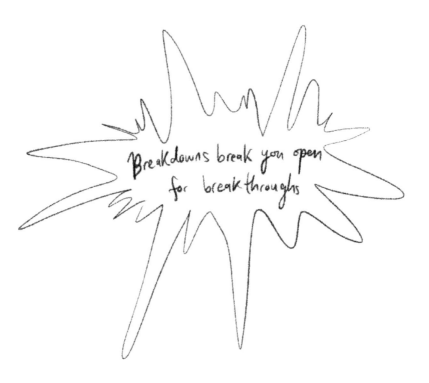

Breakdowns break you open
for breakthroughs

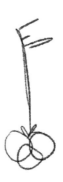

Awakening

If your life was a book
and this current chapter
came to an end

how
would
the next one
begin?

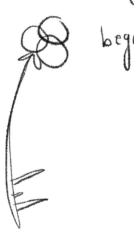

Awakening

It's not <u>what</u>
you
do

but

<u>how</u>
you
do
it
that
matters.

Awakening

The past and future are only thoughts

The only reality is <u>now</u>

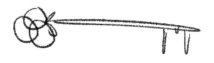

Awakening

Everything you see, everything you
touch, everyone you meet, serves
as contrast to show you
what you're _not_, and in
knowing what you're not
you can find out what
you _are_.

Awakening

Look behind your:
→ thoughts
→ fears
→ possessions
→ beliefs
→ relationships
and deep within you
you'll hear
your
heart's voice
* oh so quiet *
but
* oh so present *

Awakening

You're not "crazy." You see beyond what others can comprehend. You don't fit the status quo. And that's a good thing.

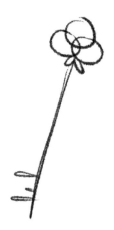

Awakening

There is no <u>one</u>
right way to be.

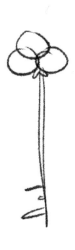

Awakening

Each note, each individual, plays an important role in the orchestra of life.

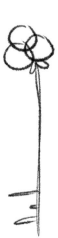

Awakening

How can you tune your instrument if you aren't willing to make a sound?

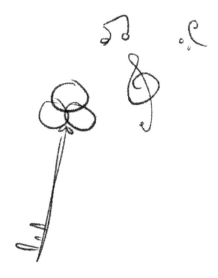

Awakening

Behind every pair
of eyes is a soul
wanting to be
loved and wanting
to love.

Awakening

Humans only
see 5% of the
universe

To think anyone knows
all there is to know
about anything is
quite preposterous!

Awakening

Giving from the mind is always conditional

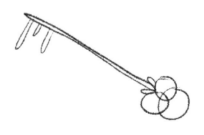

Unconditional giving can only come from the heart

Awakening

Life doesn't happen to you, it happens _for_ you.

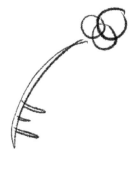

Awakening

If you
close yourself
off to
the world,
how do
you
expect
to
receive
anything?

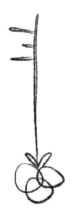

Awakening

You don't
owe
anyone
anything.

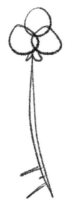

Awakening

Money is the middle-man
in the exchange of love

And love, like
money, flows most
abundantly to you
when you give
most abundantly.

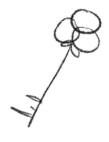

Awakening

When you stop listening
you stop being free.

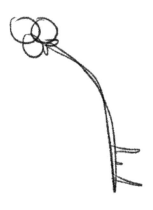

Awakening

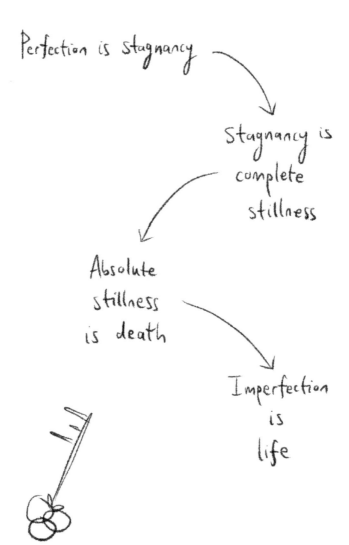

Perfection is stagnancy

Stagnancy is complete stillness

Absolute stillness is death

Imperfection is life

Awakening

I am grateful
for
<u>everything</u>
because I know
what it feels like
to not have
<u>anything</u>

Awakening

You are an
extraordinary soul
experiencing itself
through an ordinary
human form

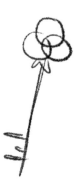

Awakening

You can both
honor the past
and not indulge
in things that no
longer serve you

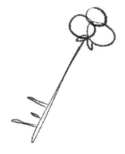

Just because it was
discarded doesn't
mean it lacks
value

Remember that everything
in the trash served a
purpose too

Awakening

Are you willing to be a kid again in the playground of life?

To know that there's a lot that you don't know and keep going?

To find pleasure in the simplest things?

To be curious and open-minded to what the playground has to offer?

Awakening

You never
regret acting out
of love.

Awakening

Every single
person is an
extension of
you.

You are an
extension of
life.

We are all
one.

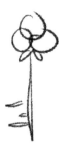

Awakening

Surrendering to aliveness doesn't mean you stop doing

If that was the case then this book wouldn't exist!

It just means *being* comes before doing

And *doing* comes from inspiration

No force is needed

161

Awakening

You're not late.

You're right on time.

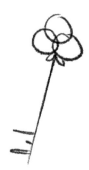

Awakening

What
you
- spot -
you
got

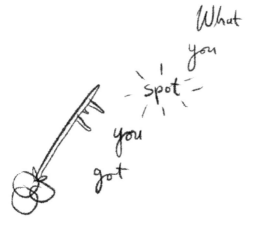

Awakening

There is absolutely
nothing I
would change about
you

but that's no excuse to
stay complacent
because
complacency is not who you are.

You are an everchanging, constantly
flowing part of life.

Awakening

The part of you
that resonates with
my writing is the
part of you that
already knows
that I don't
bring new
answers.

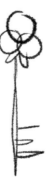

All I do
is help you
remember
what you
already
know.

Awakening

True love isn't chaotic

It isn't a rollercoaster of emotions

It feels right

It feels natural

It feels still

Awakening

I'm not willing
to settle because
I know what I'm
worth.

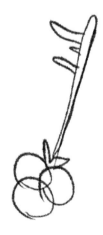

Awakening

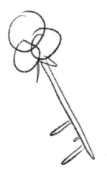

The answers
are always simple.
If they are
complex, then
they are not the
truth.

Awakening

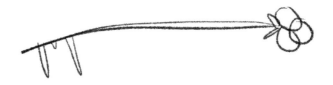

The more you know the more you
realize that you don't know.
But, who really knows?

Awakening

Question
what
I
say
for
I (the translator)

am
only

human

too
.
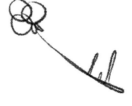

Awakening

Just like a seed
you need time
to germinate, time
to develop. Slow

phases are
most essential
in the production
of healthy
flowers.

Be patient.

In time, you will bloom.

Awakening

Seeds grow in the dark

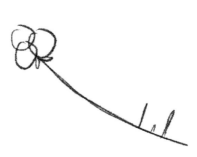

Awakening

Respect the ground from which you walk.
Respect the trees which give you air.
Respect the water from which you cleanse.
Respect the planet which gives you life.

For without them, there wouldn't be us.

Awakening

You are as beautiful as
the Milky Way

Sparkling brightly from

within

Awakening

Work doesn't feel like work

when it comes the from heart.

Awakening

What would it feel like
for your inner child to
take over for a day?

To let yourself
roam free

♡

♡

To let yourself
play

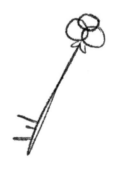

Awakening

You are only responsible
for your own emotions
for you quite literally
cannot control what
goes on in someone else's
mind.

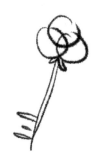

Awakening

The quality of the step
that you take right now
determines the
quality of where you
arrive.

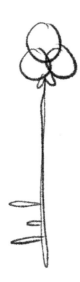

Awakening

True freedom
is the ability to
let go of blame
(towards yourself
and towards others)

Awakening

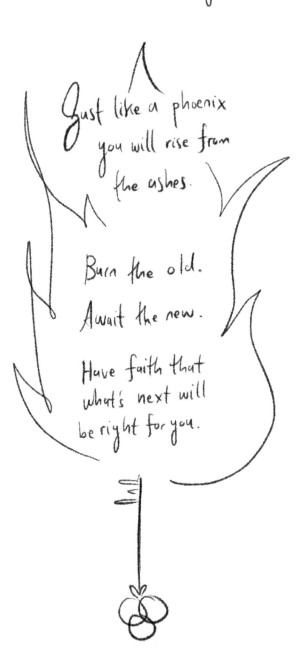

Just like a phoenix
you will rise from
the ashes.

Burn the old.
Await the new.

Have faith that
what's next will
be right for you.

Awakening

If it's not a

= fuck yes =

then what's missing?

What is it you're fearing?

Awakening

Only the truth will set 👀 you 👀 free!

Awakening

I create
everything
from
nothing

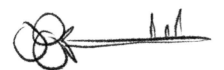

Awakening

If I can do it,
so can you

for the
part of me
that does
things

is human
too.

Awakening

Be mindful of role models —
they may have qualities
that you admire,
but you have
qualities that they'd
admire. Your role models
serve a unique role
and so do you.
Don't lose sight of
your gifts.

Awakening

We are all made
of star dust

There's light
in every one of
us

Will you
let yours
shine?

186

Awakening

It took billions of years
for this present moment to
become a reality. Everything —
all life, lessons, creations —
has brought today into
fruition.

Pretty miraculous, right?!

Awakening

Whatever you do,
experience it fully

how else will
you know that it
was the most aligned
thing to do?

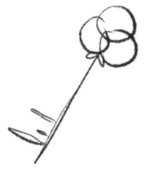

Awakening

If you need
a break, take
a break

If you want
to bake a pie,
bake a pie

If you want
to dress up,
dress up

Just because you've become more conscious of habits in your life doesn't mean everything needs to be perfectly aligned at the snap of a finger. It's the intention that matters, not the accuracy.

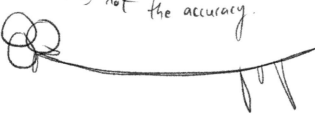

Awakening

Taking personal responsibility
doesn't mean seeing
yourself as the problem
every time you
experience pain.

It means honoring your
natural human needs
for love, safety,
and belonging —
knowing when or how
to ask for or give them
to yourself.

Awakening

You can't hold
space for others
when your
container is
weak

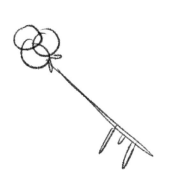

Weak containers
that hold more
than they can
carry break or
leak.

Awakening

Sometimes the wisest
thing to do is nothing
at all.

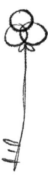

Awakening

I'll be honest...

    you will be misunderstood

    you will feel lonely

    you will mess up

    you will face criticism

    you will have to make tough choices

And at the same time...

    you are not alone

    you are loved

    you are significant

    you are beautiful

    you are more than enough

    you are free

Awakening

In silence
and stillness
you can hear
your soul's

wh
i
s
p
e
r.

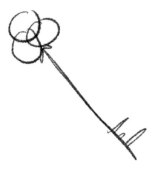

Awakening

You just might find
treasures handed to
you because they are
exactly what you
want and what the
other person doesn't
value any more. Exchanges
can be that easy

(and mutually gratifying)!

Awakening

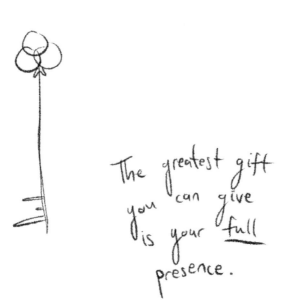

The greatest gift
you can give
is your <u>full</u>
presence.

Awakening

The secret ingredient
behind all of your
greatest creations
is *you*.

Awakening

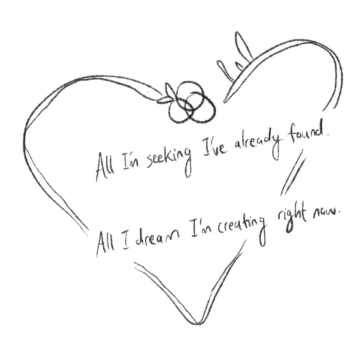

All I'm seeking I've already found.

All I dream I'm creating right now.

Awakening

There's nothing (no _thing_)
that can bring
you happiness but you

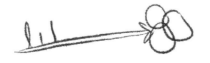

Awakening

Falling
deeper
and
deeper
into
the
mental void
which feels endless
you will
get to
the
bottom
and
actually
find
the
key

It had been there
all along

Awakening

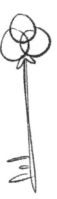

Open your heart
and you will find
all you wish for
is there inside.

Awakening

There is never a need to shove
a message down anyone's throat

If they are curious,
they will ask

and if they
don't, it's <u>not</u> their loss

it may not
be the right time
or it may not be
the right person.

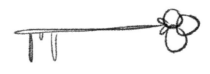

Awakening

There is no point after-all... so why not have some fun?

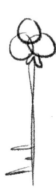

Awakening

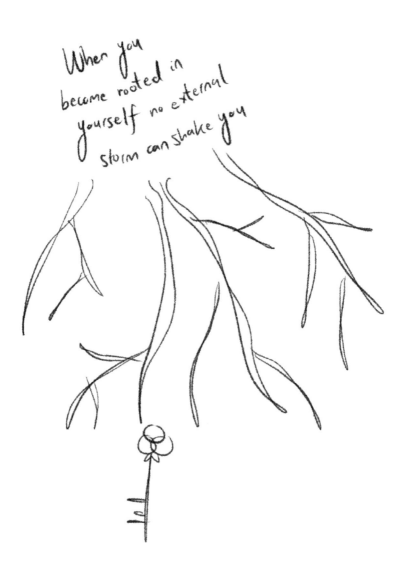

When you become rooted in yourself no external storm can shake you

Awakening

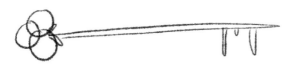

Slow
down.

Life
is
not
to
be
rushed,
it's
to
be
lived .

Awakening

Just because you
found your key
doesn't mean you
have the secret
formula. The path
to discovery is
different for everyone.

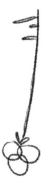

Awakening

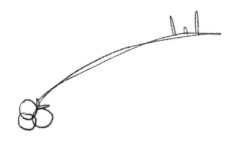

Sometimes there's no
easy way to explain
reality, and sometimes
reality is not meant to
be explained.

Feel for yourself
what's energetically
true for you. That's
all you really need.

Awakening

You know you've changed when
what used to startle you then
has little effect on you
now.

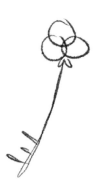

Awakening

You're in a human vehicle

It's only natural to have human desires

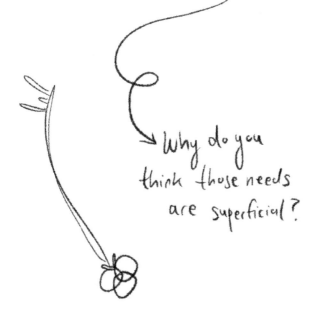

Why do you think those needs are superficial?

209

Awakening

It's okay to have discovered your
power and to have tasted freedom,
now only to find yourself back
in your cage. You always have
another opportunity to break
free, and now at least
you know you
can.

Awakening

Find your center.

Breathe into that space.

Ground yourself.

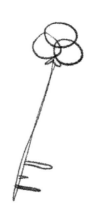

Awakening

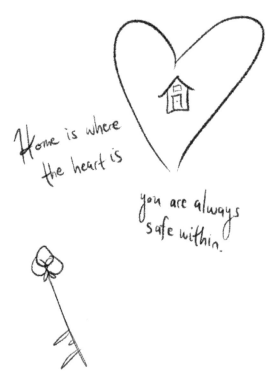

Home is where
the heart is

you are always
safe within.

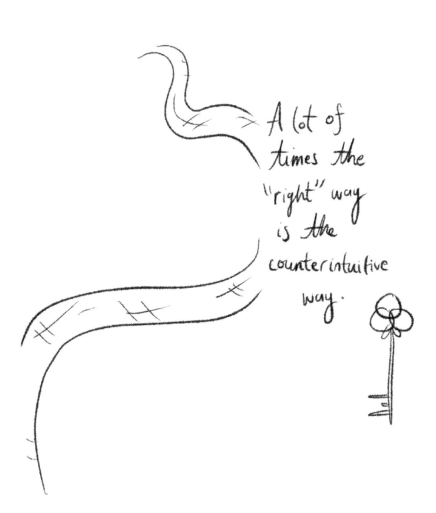

A lot of times the "right" way is the counterintuitive way.

Awakening

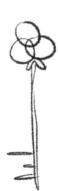

The gift
is in the

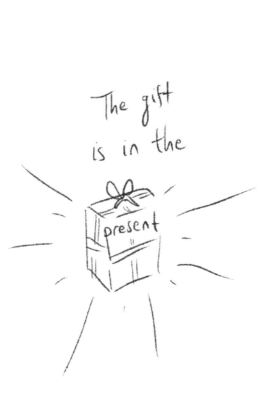

present

Without you life is
incomplete.

You are the
missing puzzle
piece.

Awakening

All is right

All is well

All is complete.

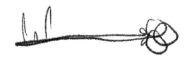

About The Author

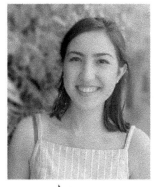

Hi! I'm Anna, an ICF Certified Life Coach with additional experience as a Software Engineer, Product Manager, and elementary school instructor. I describe myself as a truth seeker, lover of life, adventurer, and artist. My simple view of life is that everything can be done in either love or fear. Some of my deepest values include being honest and true to yourself, loving yourself first, living consciously, and inspiring through embodiment. I believe that every soul is here for a reason and that the physical material in our human experience is material for us to return back to know ourselves. I feel that at the core of everything is love.

Website: intentionallyanna.com
Inquiries: anna@intentionallyanna.com
Instagram: @intentionallyanna